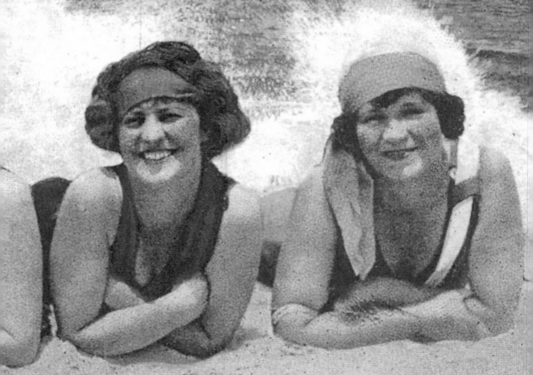

Bathing Beauties
of the Roaring '20s

Mary L. Martin
Tina Skinner

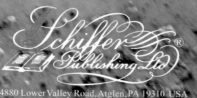

Schiffer Publishing Ltd ®

4880 Lower Valley Road, Atglen, PA 19310 USA

About the Authors

Mary Martin Postcards is a three-generation family business and the largest postcard operation in the world. In addition to a warehouse facility in Perryville, Maryland, the company is a presence at postcard shows worldwide, and produces many shows, including the nation's largest postcard show in York, Pennsylvania, in November. They are located at www.marylmartin.com and can be telephoned at 410-642-3581. Tina Skinner is a professional writer and editor.

Published by Schiffer Publishing Ltd.
4880 Lower Valley Road
Atglen, PA 19310
Phone: (610) 593-1777;
Fax: (610) 593-2002
E-mail: Info@schifferbooks.com

For the largest selection of fine reference books on this and related subjects, please visit our web site at
www.schifferbooks.com
We are always looking for people to write books on new and related subjects. If you have an idea for a book please contact us at the above address.

This book may be purchased from the publisher.
Include $3.95 for shipping.
Please try your bookstore first.
You may write for a free catalog.

In Europe, Schiffer books are distributed by
Bushwood Books
6 Marksbury Ave.
Kew Gardens
Surrey TW9 4JF England
Phone: 44 (0) 20 8392-8585;
Fax: 44 (0) 20 8392-9876
E-mail: info@bushwoodbooks.co.uk
Free postage in the U.K., Europe;
air mail at cost.

Copyright © 2005 by Mary L. Martin
Library of Congress Card Number: 2004107479

Type set in Humanist 521 BT/Humanist 521 BT

ISBN: 0-7643-2116-1
Printed in China

Introduction

Fashions changed radically in the 1920s, and so did women. In redefining their role in society, women also radically altered their outwear, from full skirts that swept the floor, to straight sheaths that stopped short of shins. This didn't change when they headed out on holiday. The modest, full-bodied hosiery and dress swimwear of earlier eras was shed in favor of body hugging half-suits. Shoulders emerged along with the shins, and a lot more skin experienced the sun than ever enjoyed the light of day during the relatively stuffy Victorian era.

However, you're not going to find sleazy or overly suggestive images herein. Instead, you'll find refreshing, energetic exposures, shared on sunny, happy vacations. Travel vicariously back in time with shore-side shutterbugs as they flattered their shapely subjects and helped them feel pretty. You'll be charmed.

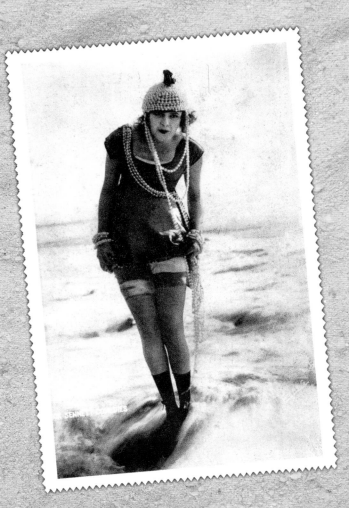

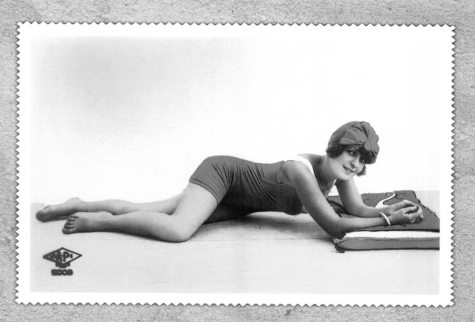

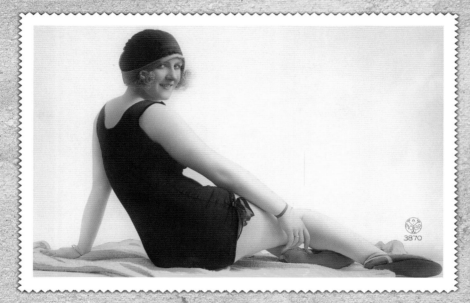

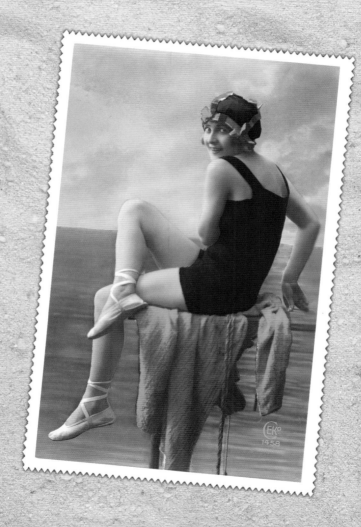

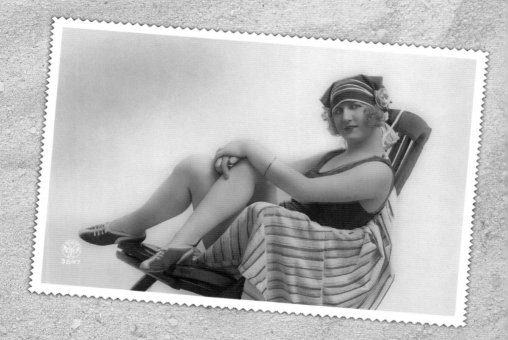

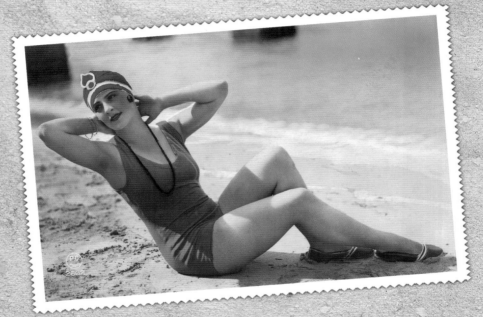

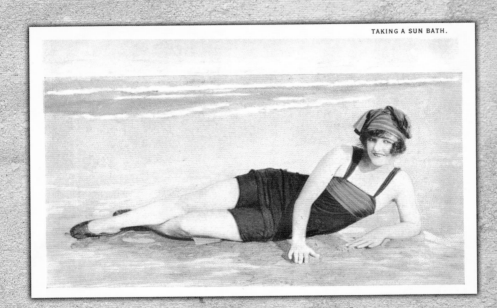

TAKING A SUN BATH.

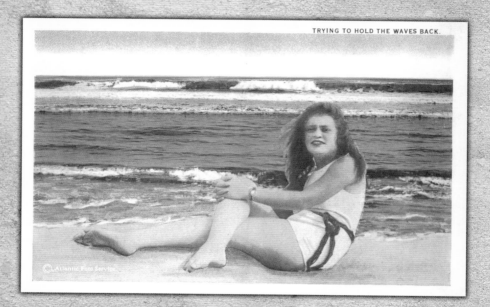

TRYING TO HOLD THE WAVES BACK.

© Atlantic Foto Service

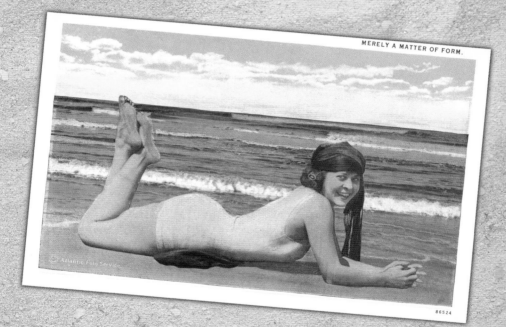

MERELY A MATTER OF FORM.

© Atlantic Foto Service

86524

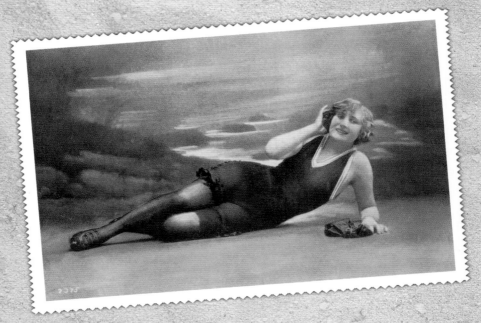

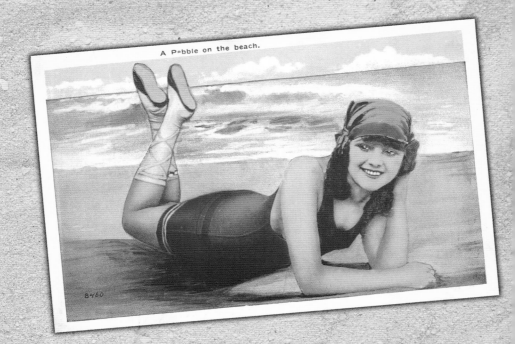

A Pebble on the beach.

8460

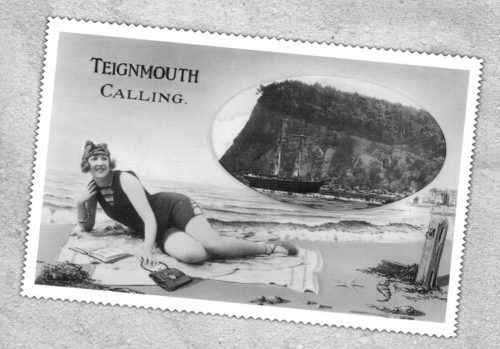

TEIGNMOUTH
CALLING.

NESS ROCK AND ENTRANCE TO RIVER TEIGN

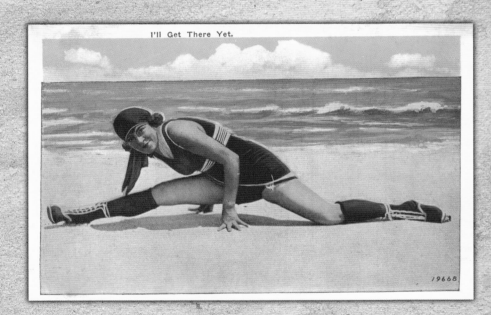

I'll Get There Yet.

19668

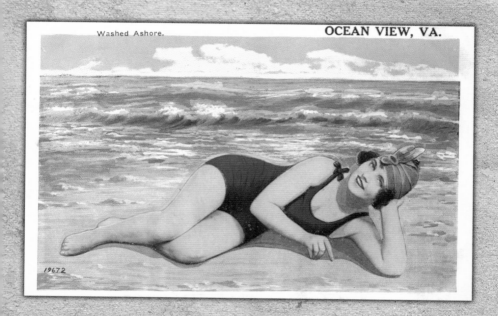

Washed Ashore.

OCEAN VIEW, VA.

19672

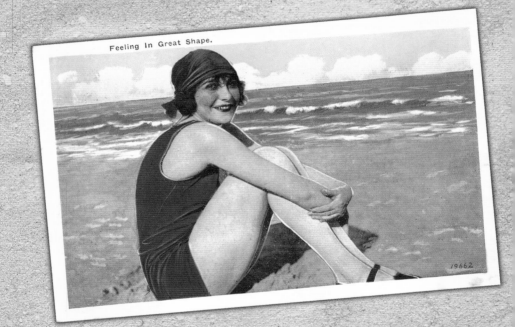

Feeling In Great Shape.

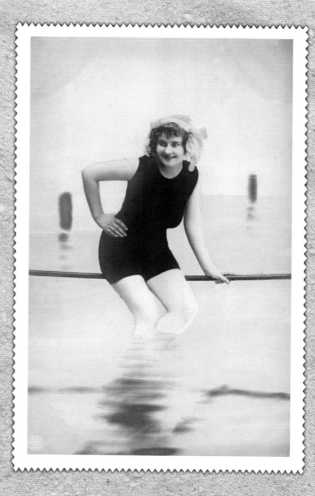

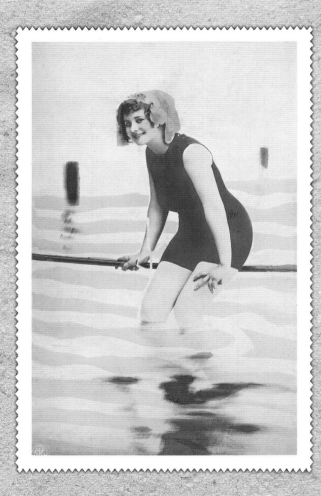

Having My Hands Full Here.

OCEAN VIEW, VA.

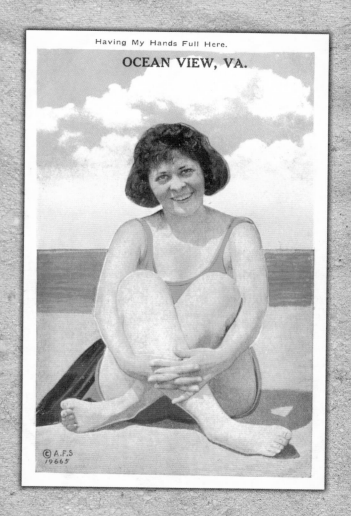

© A.F.S
19665

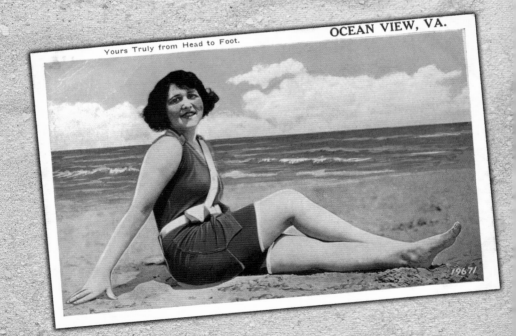

Yours Truly from Head to Foot.

OCEAN VIEW, VA.

19671

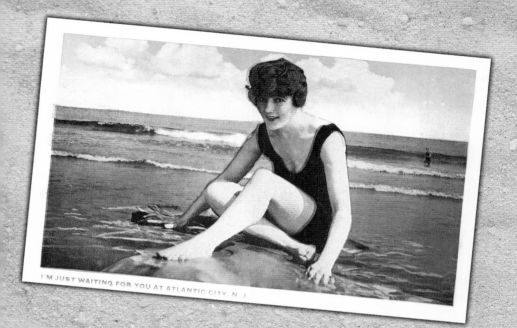

I'M JUST WAITING FOR YOU AT ATLANTIC CITY, N. J.

How would you like to be here

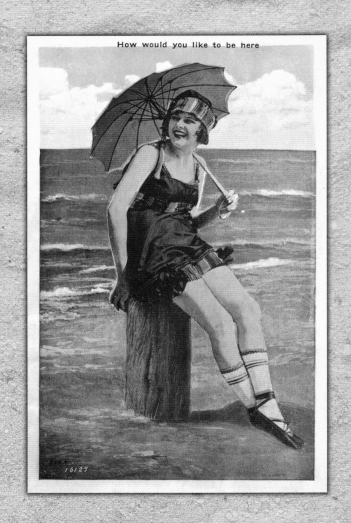

16125

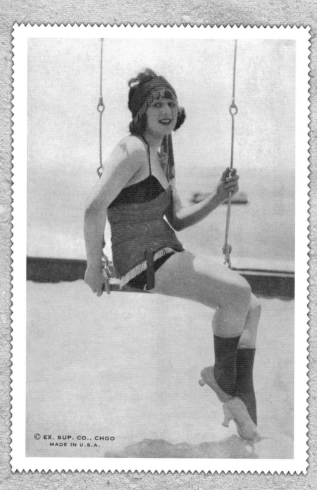

© EX. SUP. CO., CHGO
MADE IN U.S.A.

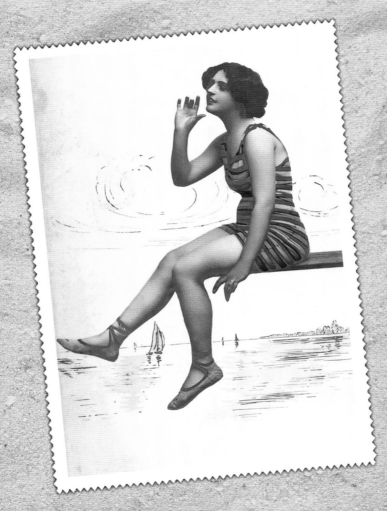

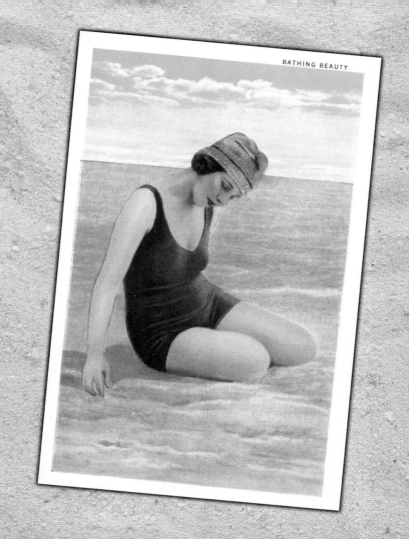

BATHING BEAUTY.

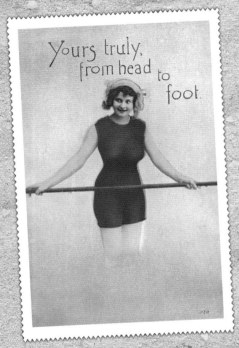

Yours truly,
from head to foot.

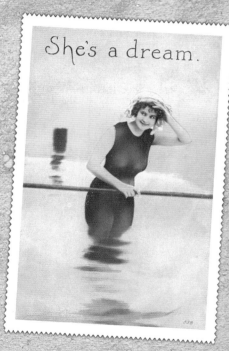

She's a dream.

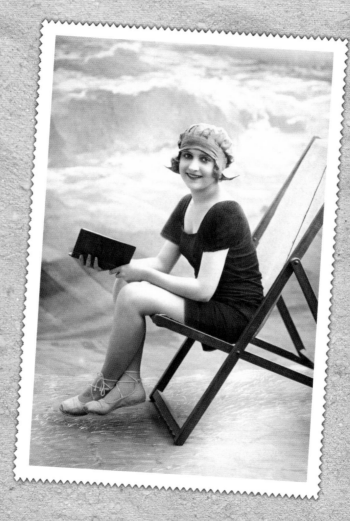

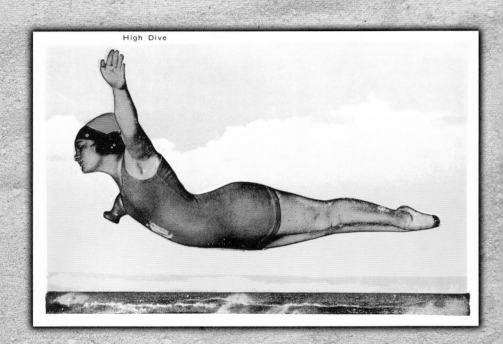

High Dive

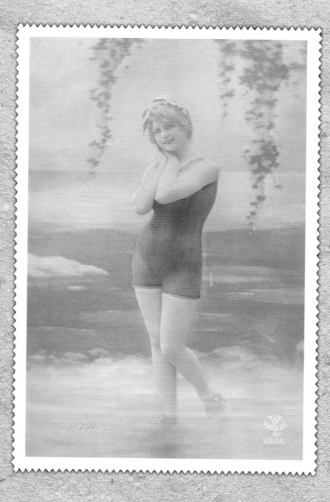

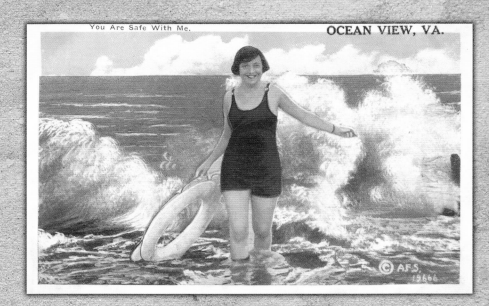

You Are Safe With Me.

OCEAN VIEW, VA.

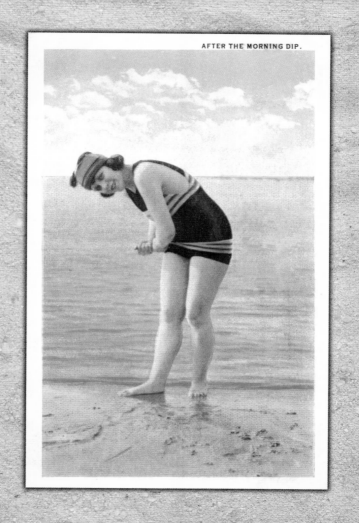

AFTER THE MORNING DIP.

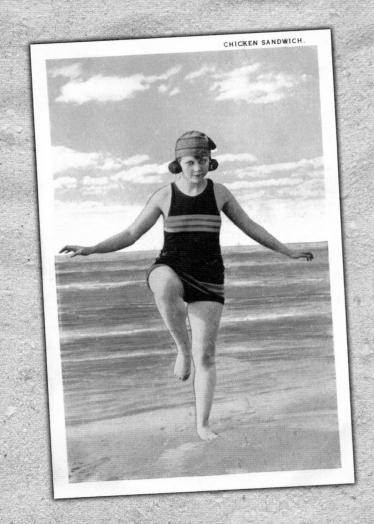

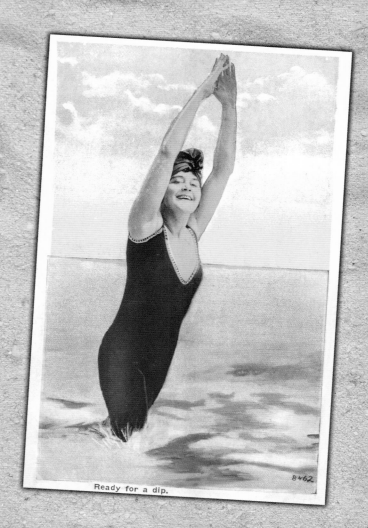

Ready for a dip.

8462

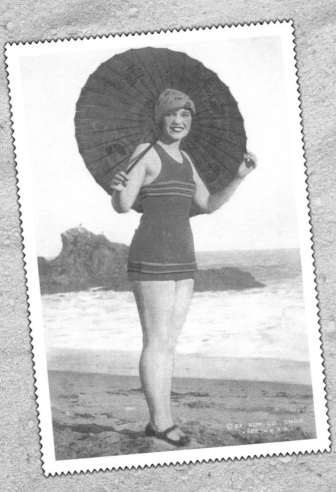

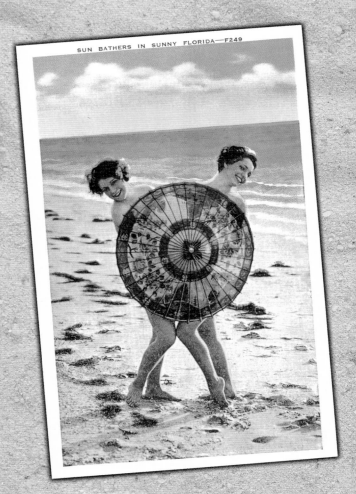

SUN BATHERS IN SUNNY FLORIDA—F249

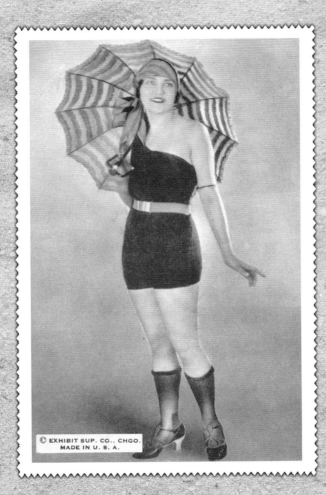

© EXHIBIT SUP. CO., CHGO.
MADE IN U. S. A.

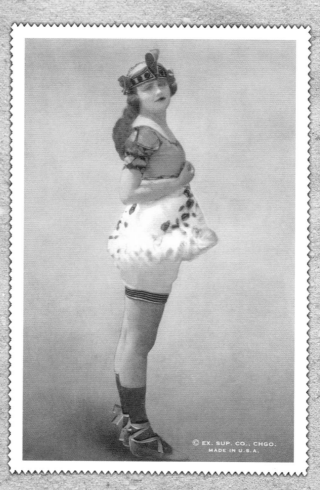

© EX. SUP. CO., CHGO.
MADE IN U.S.A.

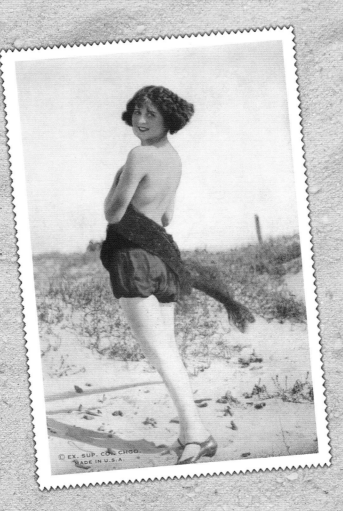

© EX. SUP. CO., CHGO.
MADE IN U.S.A.

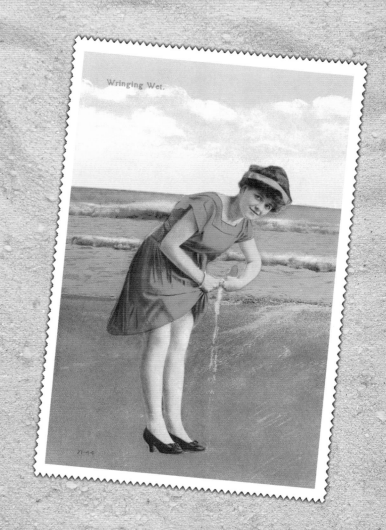

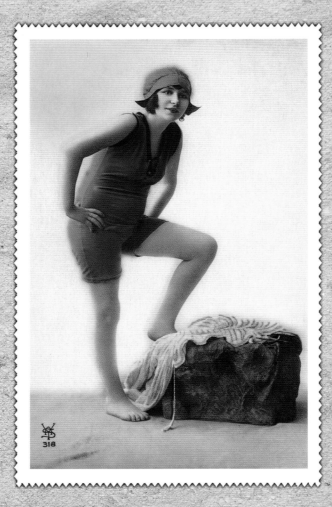

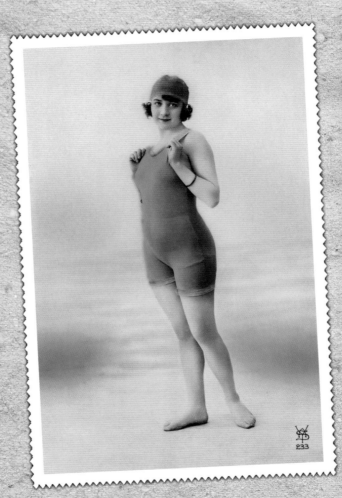

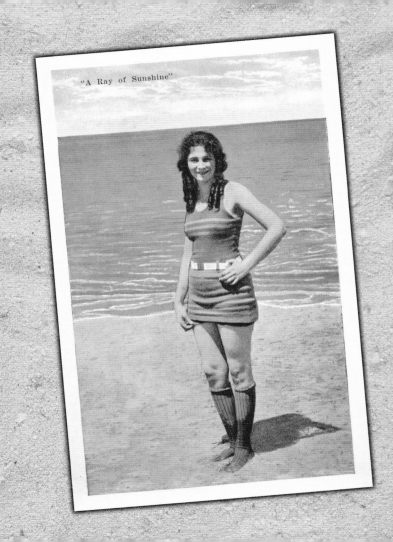

"A Ray of Sunshine"

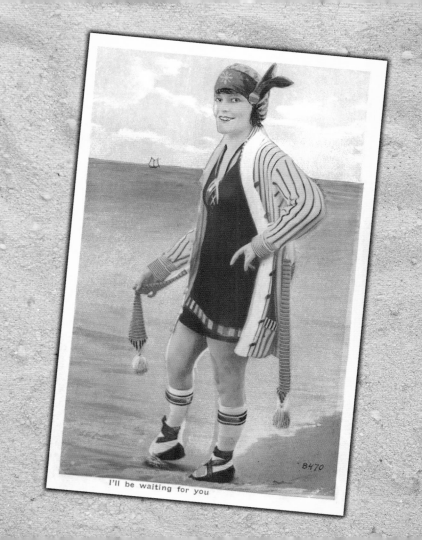

I'll be waiting for you

8470

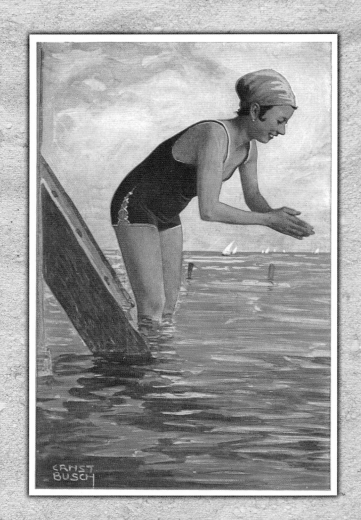

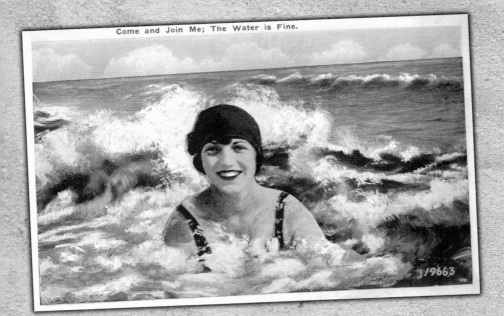

Come and Join Me; The Water is Fine.

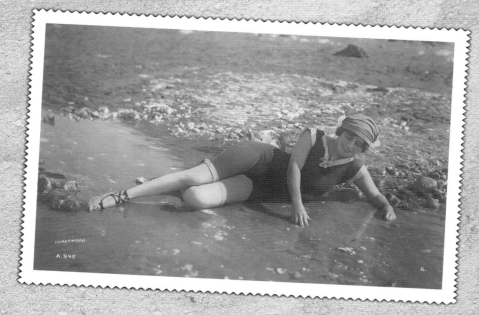

UNDERWOOD.

A.942

6.

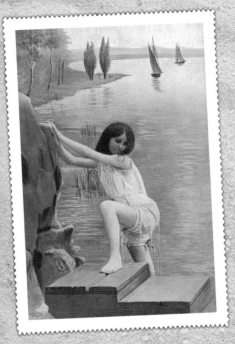

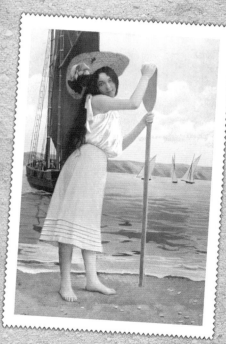

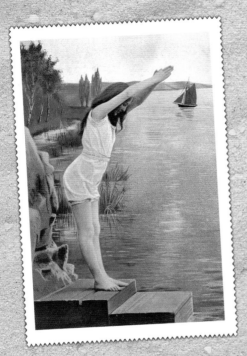
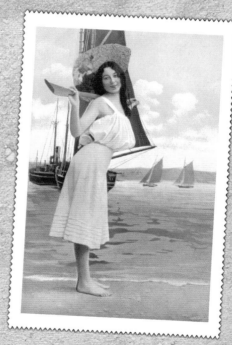

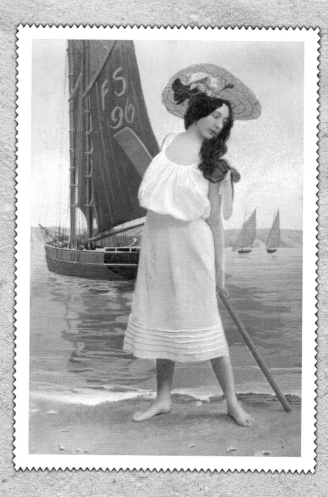

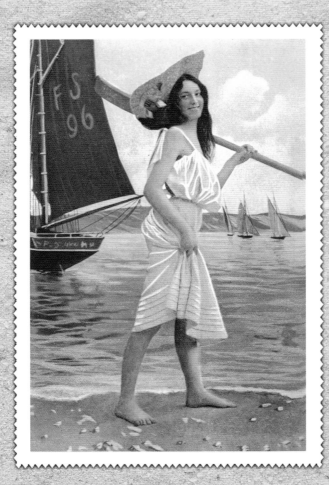

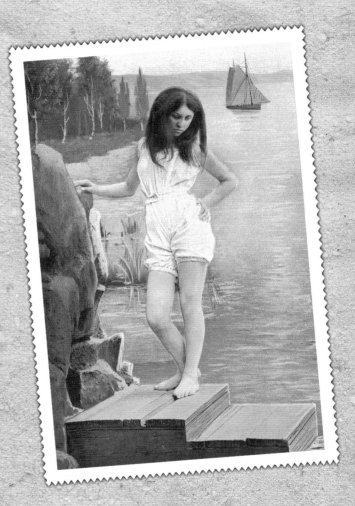

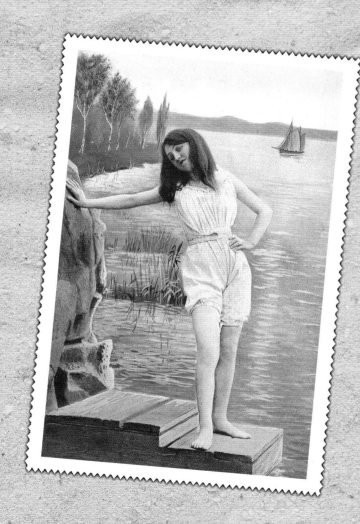

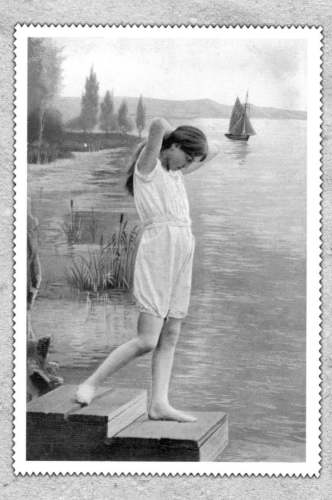

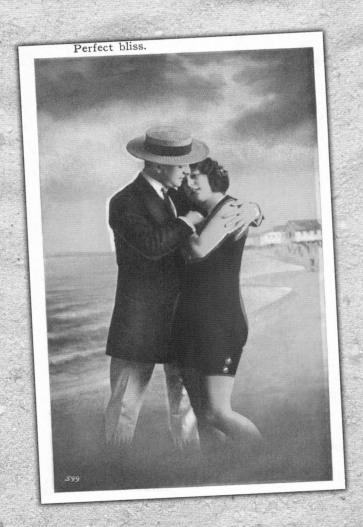

Perfect bliss.

599

A summer pastime.

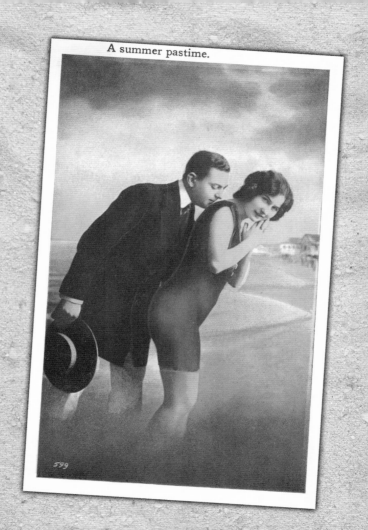

599

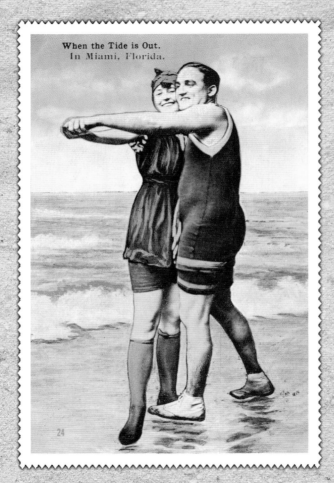

When the Tide is Out.
In Miami, Florida.

24

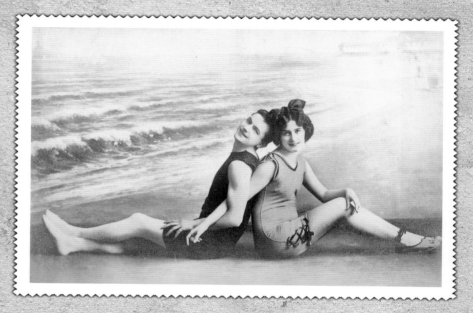

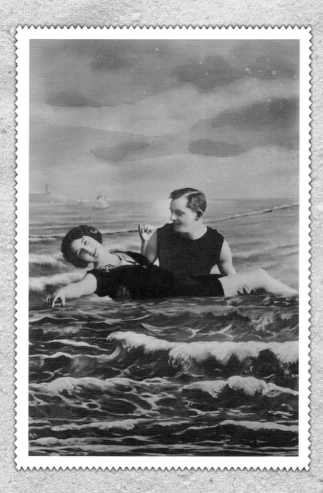

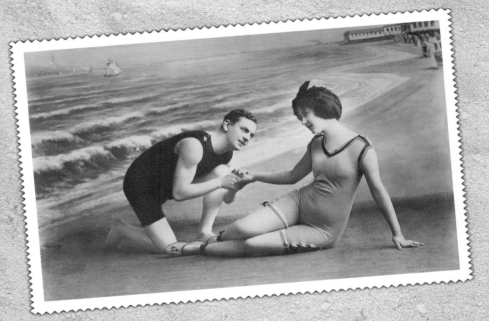

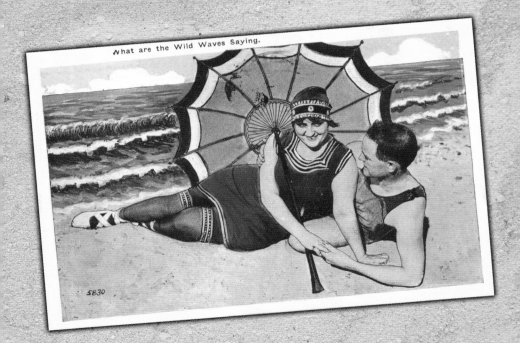

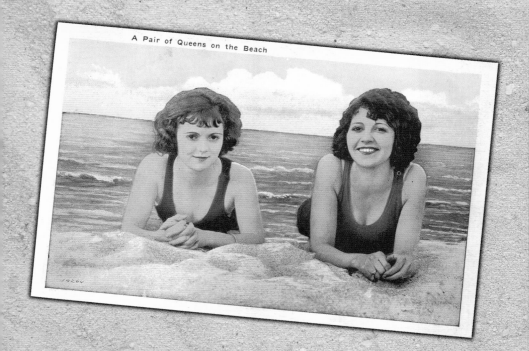

A Pair of Queens on the Beach

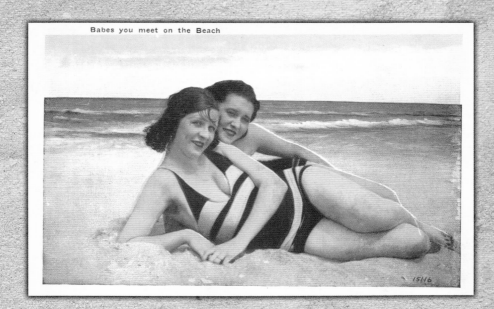

Babes you meet on the Beach

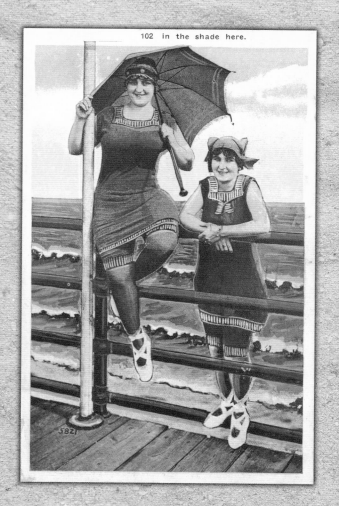

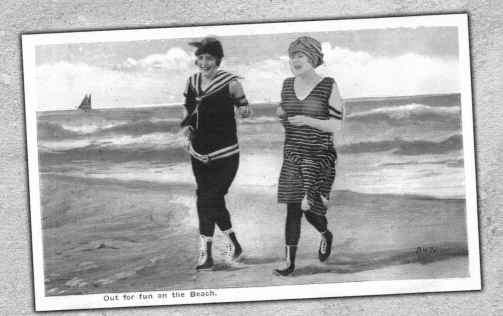

Out for fun on the Beach.

8471

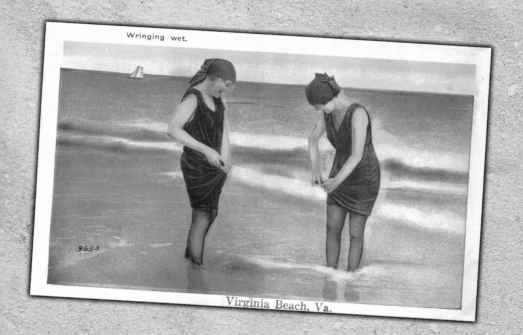

Wringing wet.

9653

Virginia Beach, Va.

"Peek-a-boo". Me for You

536

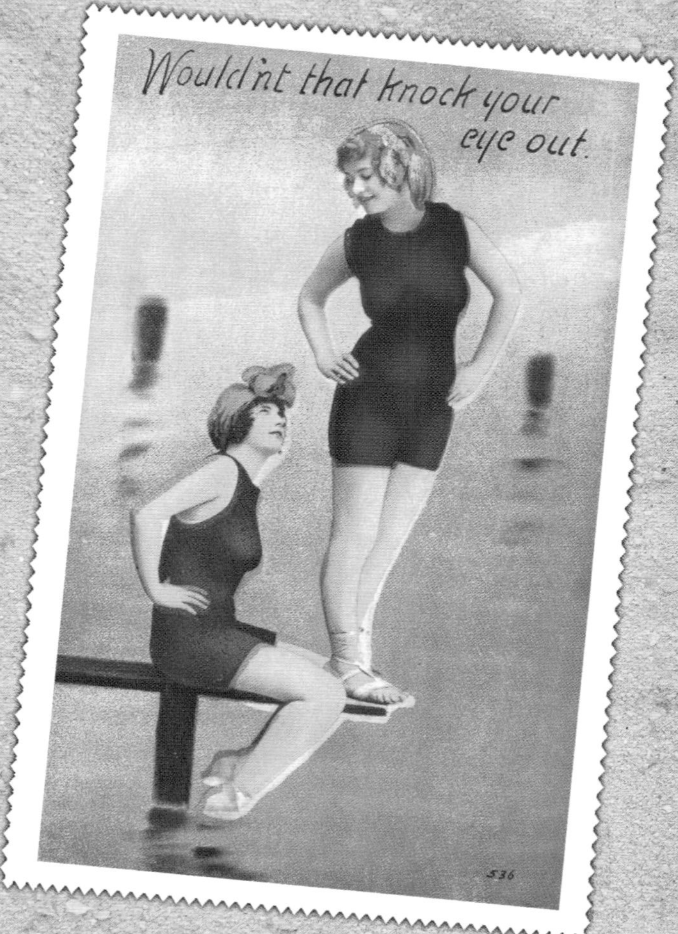
Would'nt that knock your eye out.
536

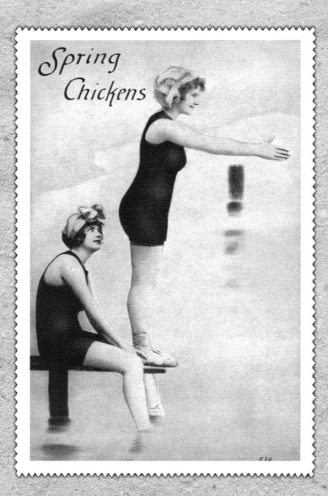

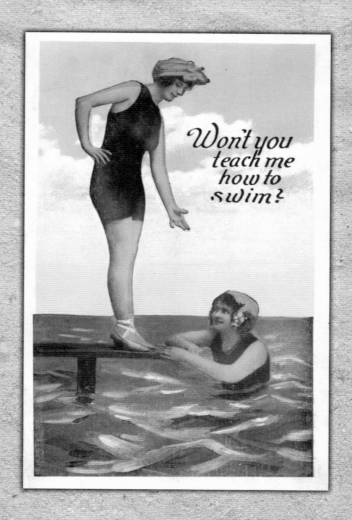

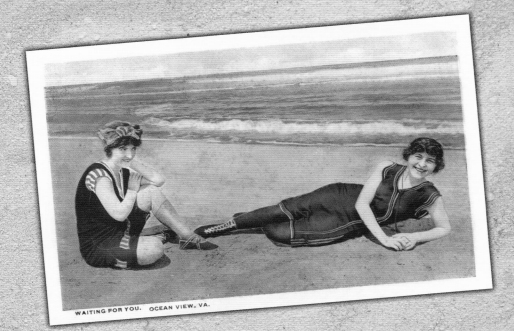

WAITING FOR YOU.   OCEAN VIEW, VA.

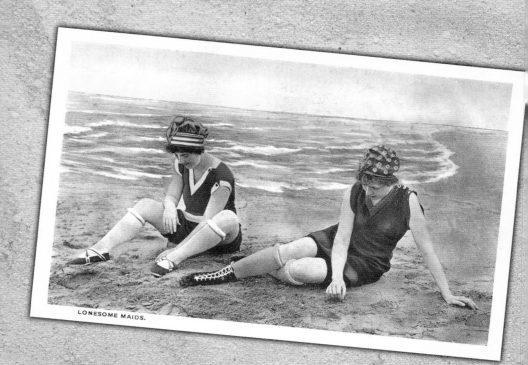

LONESOME MAIDS.

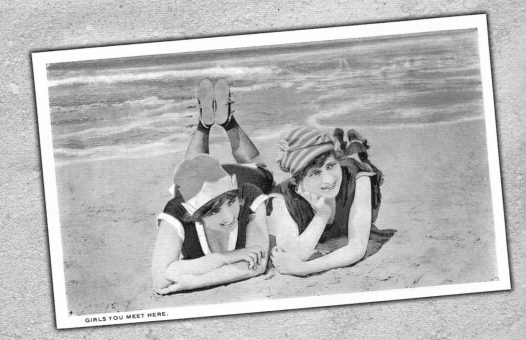

GIRLS YOU MEET HERE.

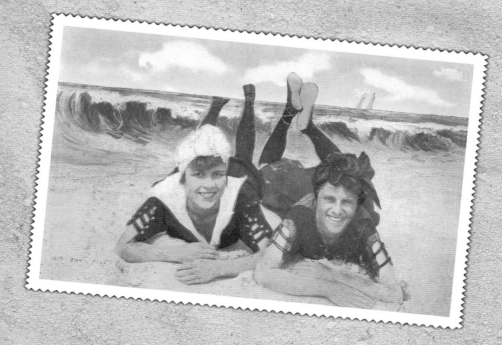

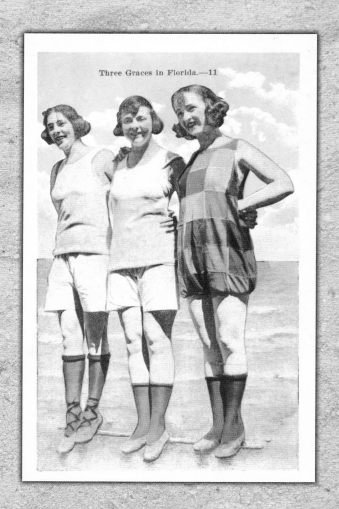

Three Graces in Florida.—11

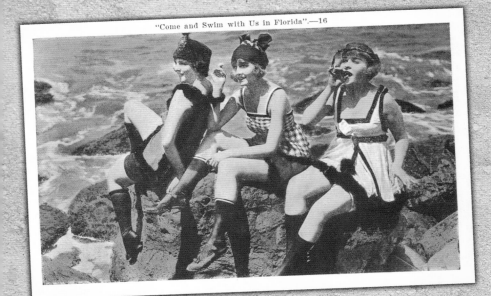

"Come and Swim with Us in Florida".—16

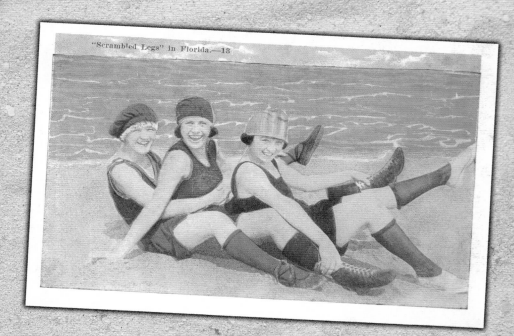

"Scrambled Legs" in Florida.—13

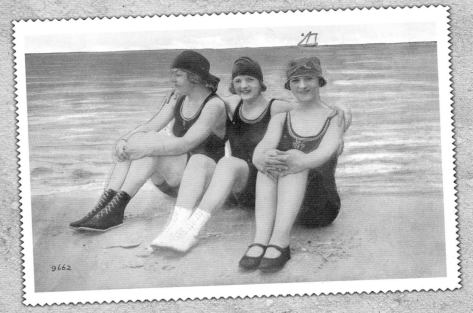

9662

I'm taking my annual

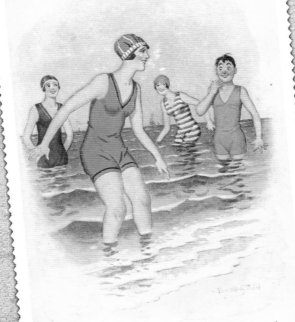

Don't forget to take your annual.

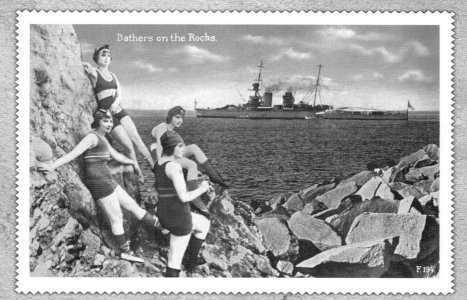

Bathers on the Rocks.

F.194

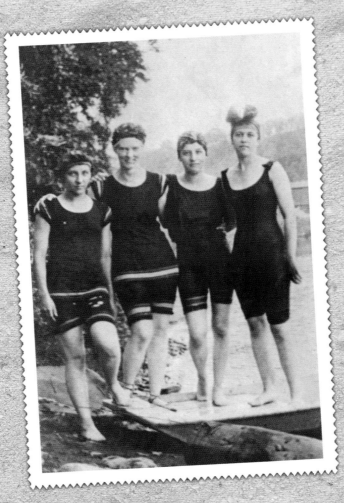

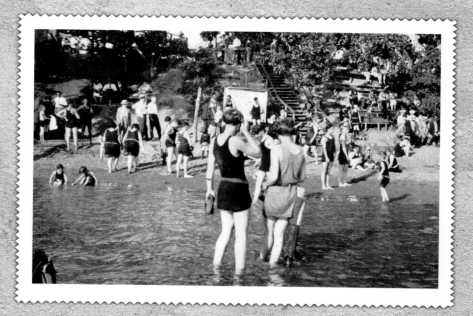

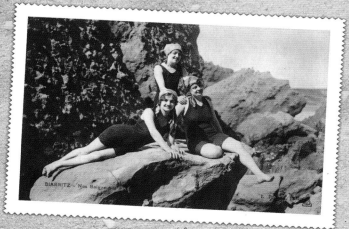

BIARRITZ - Nos Baigneuses

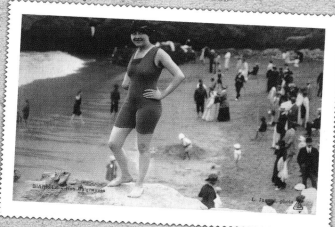

BIARRITZ - Nos Baigneuses

L. Jusseau, photo

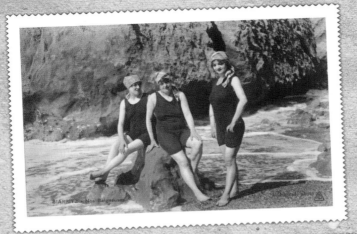

BIARRITZ – Nos Baigneuses

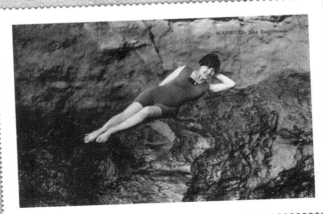

BIARRITZ – Nos Baigneuses

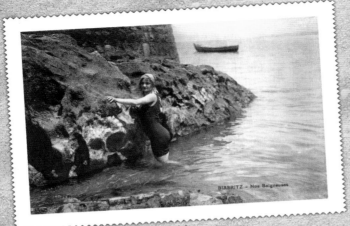

BIARRITZ – Nos Baigneuses

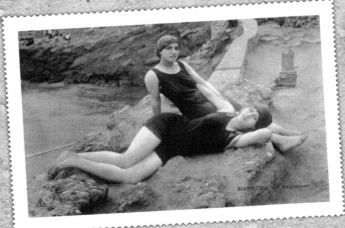

BIARRITZ – Nos Baigneuses

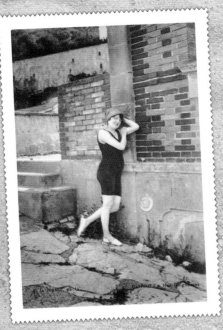

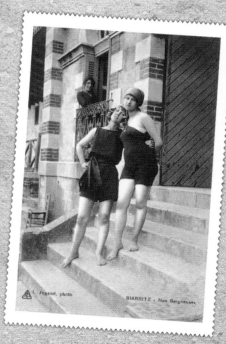

BIARRITZ - Nos Baigneuses

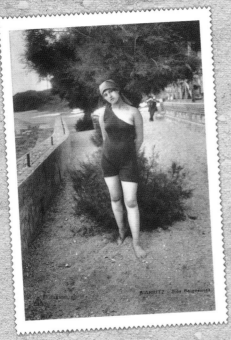

BIARRITZ - Nos Baigneuses

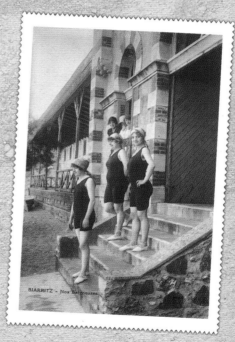

BIARRITZ - Nos Baigneuses

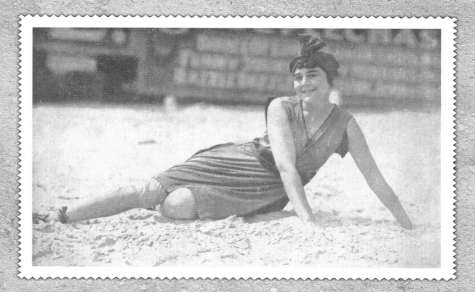

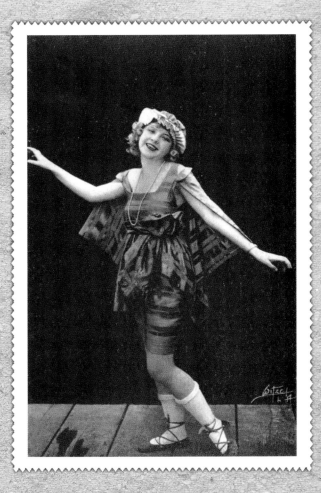

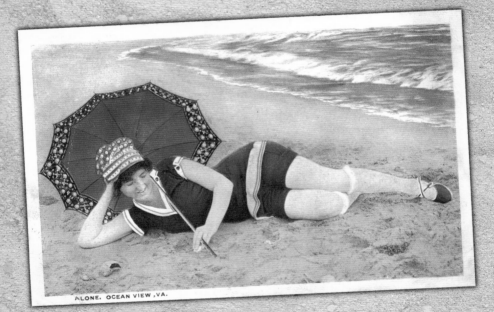

ALONE. OCEAN VIEW ,VA.

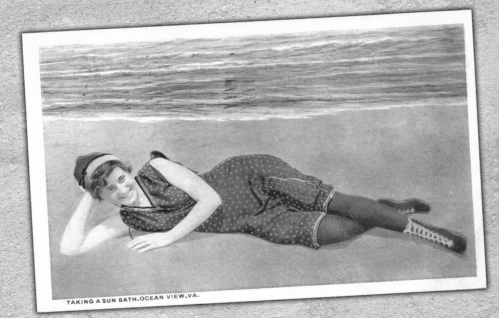

TAKING A SUN BATH, OCEAN VIEW, VA.

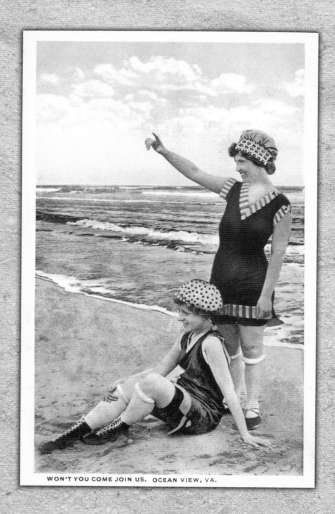

WON'T YOU COME JOIN US. OCEAN VIEW, VA.

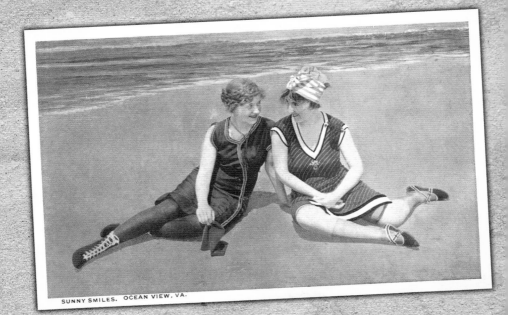

SUNNY SMILES. OCEAN VIEW, VA.

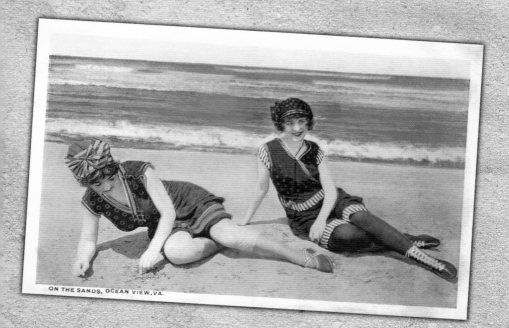

ON THE SANDS, OCEAN VIEW, VA.

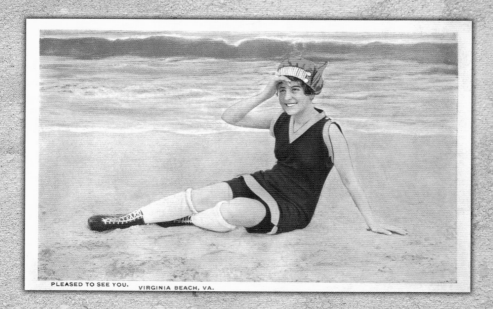

PLEASED TO SEE YOU.   VIRGINIA BEACH, VA.